## Related Kaplan Books

EMT-Basic Exam

KAPLAN

# EMS Flashcards

Compiled by Richard J. Lapierre

Simon & Schuster

New York · London · Sydney · Toronto

Kaplan Publishing
Published by SIMON & SCHUSTER
Rockefeller Center
1230 Avenue of the Americas
New York, NY 10020



Editorial Director: Jennifer Farthing

Project Editor: Cynthia C. Yazbek

Production Manager: Michael Shevlin

Content Manager: Patrick Kennedy

Interior Page Layout: Dave Chipps

Cover Design: Mark Weaver

Manufactured in the United States of America
Published simultaneously in Canada

10 9 8 7 6 5 4 3 2 1

October 2005

ISBN-13: 978-0-7432-7874-4

ISBN-10: 0-7432-7874-7

For information regarding special discounts for bulk purchases, please contact Simon & Schuster Special Sales at 1-800-456-6798 or business@simonandschuster.com.

# How to Use This Book

This book provides an easy way to remember the terms and values necessary to function as an EMS professional, healthcare worker, or first-responder. Simply read the item name on the front of the flashcard; then flip the page for the correct answer. This will help you remember and reinforce the knowledge you've already gained in your courses and it will help you to prepare for the licensing exam.

We've divided these into the following categories:

- Acronyms
- Medications
- Anatomy
    - Descriptions of the Body
    - Bones
    - Organs
    - Muscles

- Normal Vital Signs
    * Adult
    * Pediatric
    * Infant
- Medical/Legal Terminology
- Pediatric Terms
- Medical Equipment
- Truck Check Items
- Treatment Modalities
- Which Protocol?

After you correctly answer one of the pages, you can either fold the corner of the page or place a paper clip on it so when you review again you can skip right over it.

This book contains a lot of information and once you've read it from front to back, you can turn it over and find another set of terms and values reading from back to front.

At the conclusion of the categories is a chapter entitled "Which Protocol?" that presents you with a scenario and challenges you to determine "which protocol" you have learned applies to that scene. This provides you with a way to pull together all that you have learned in class to prepare for the licensing exam.

In pre-hospital emergency medicine, doing one's best is of the utmost importance, because medical professionals and first-responders deal with life and death issues every day. Those of us engaged in teaching this important discipline take it very seriously, and wish to impart the best methods of learning the discipline upon you, our students, so that when you engage in practice you will be among the best purveyors of this craft.

All of us here at Kaplan wish you the best as you prepare to begin your career as a first-responder. We are confident that these tools will help you prepare yourself to save lives each day.

Good luck!

Note to the reader:

This book is authorized for use as a study aid for preparation for an EMT, first responder, firefighter, or other emergency medical service-related certification exams only. Kaplan is not liable for any uses other than as a study aid. For on-the-job resources, please consult board-approved information.

## Fractured Clavicle

To properly splint a fractured clavicle, secure the patient's arm on the affected side with a sling to support the lower arm and tie a wide swath bandage across the chest to hold the upper arm against the torso.

Acronyms

# ABC

**Airway, Breathing, Circulation:** These are the first assessment checks done to a patient. They are treated in order before moving on to any other assessments or treatments. Failure to restore these if absent is a fatal event.

**Which Protocol?**

You respond to the local high school soccer field for an injured player. You arrive on scene and find a nine-year-old male holding his right arm and complaining of pain to the area to the right of his neck. It is tender to the touch. What injury do you suspect and how do you treat it?

Acronyms

# AED

## Open Femur Fracture

The patient has an open femur fracture, which should be reduced through the use of a traction splint prior to transport.

**Automated External Defibrillator:** A device which will automatically analyze a cardiac rhythm and deliver an electrical shock in an attempt to convert a dysrhythmia to a normal rhythm.

**Which Protocol?**

You arrive at the scene of an automobile vs. bicycle accident and your patient is a 12-year-old male, lying supine with a bloody right pant leg. Your patient is conscious, alert, oriented times three, and in severe pain. You cut off the pants and you see the superior end of the patient's femur sticking out of the anterior right leg.

## Implied Consent

If you believe that the patient is incapable of making an informed decision because of hyperglycemia, then you can intervene under the legal doctrine of implied consent.

# AHA

**American Heart Association:** A national organization engaged in ongoing research and education for cardiovascular diseases. The AHA publishes standards and guidelines for CPR and ALS.

**Which Protocol?**

You respond to a call for a patient in respiratory distress. You arrive on scene and patient's mother advises you that the patient is diabetic and has not been taking her insulin on a regular basis. The patient is anxious, drooling, argumentative, and refuses to allow you to perform any interventions. She is over 18 years of age. What legal doctrine allows you to treat and transport this patient?

Acronyms

# AIDS

## Behavioral Emergency

Because of her history, you may be tempted to rush into treatment for hypoglycemia, but her blood glucose should be quickly measured with a glucometer before beginning treatment. If the patient's blood glucose level is normal, then you are left with a behavioral emergency and should transport the patient to a facility with provisions for handling mental illness.

**Acquired Immune Deficiency Syndrome:** A condition brought about by the Human Immunodeficiency Virus (see HIV) which suppresses the body's ability to fight off infections. AIDS is usually fatal.

**Which Protocol?**

You respond to a college dorm for a diabetic emergency. You arrive to find a female patient whom you have previously treated for hypoglycemia smearing feces on the hallway wall and humming to herself. Her roommate states she has been acting strangely all morning.

Acronyms

# ALS

## Behavioral Emergency

This type of restraint is dangerous and may lead to asphyxiation of the patient. EMS should immediately roll the patient on his side to remove the pressure on the patient's diaphragm. If enough personnel are present to change the patient's restraints to leather or vinyl so that the patient can be tranported supine, then that should be done. Otherwise, transport on his side with the metal restraints in place. EMS should have a key if it becomes necessary to remove the restraints to perform a medical intervention.

**Advanced Life Support:** Protocols developed by the AHA to treat various cardiac conditions by an EMT-I and EMT-P, including intravenous drugs and electrical counter shock.

**Which Protocol?**

You respond to the police station for a patient in need of transport to a medical facility. You arrive on scene and the patient is lying prone on the floor of the garage, with his hands handcuffed behind his back and his ankles cuffed together with leg irons. The chain of the leg irons is drawn up through the handcuffs so that his feet are pulled up to his hands. He is struggling violently against the restraints.

# AMI

## Behavioral Emergency

Allow the police to take this man into custody and then secure him according to your local protocols for transport to a psychiatric facility.

**Acute Myocardial Infarction:** Death of a portion of heart muscle caused by a blockage of a coronary artery. Also known as a heart attack.

**Which Protocol?**

You respond to a meet the police call at a local shopping mall. There is a bearded man, naked, proclaiming that he is a prophet and he is carrying a sign that proclaims "Drugs for All." The police officers have surrounded him and he is trying to strike them with the sign.

# APGAR SCORE

## Breech Birth

When any part other than the head of the baby presents first, this is called a breech birth and the fetus is at grave risk. Place the patient in the truck, administer oxygen, and transport priority.

**Appearance, Pulse, Grimace, Activity and Respiration:** Scoring system of signs checked at one and five minutes after childbirth. Score is a maximum of 10 and a minimum of 0.

**Which Protocol?**

You respond to a call for a woman having a baby. You arrive on scene and the woman advises you that this is her third child, that the pains began a few hours ago when her water broke, and now the pains are almost frequent. You visualize her perineum and you see a small arm protruding from the vagina.

# ARPM

## Obstetrics

These signs and symptoms are consistent with the second stage of labor. If you can visualize the baby's head during a contraction, then prepare to deliver. If not, transport priority to the nearest obstetrical hospital.

**ARPM:** Mnemonic for steps of simple triage. Ambulatory status; Respiratory status; Perfusion Status; Mental Status. Once an MCI patient is assessed for these four things, he is assigned a color and moved to the appropriate triage/treatment sector.

**Which Protocol?**

You respond to a residence for a female having abdominal pains. The patient has a large, distended abdomen and advises you that just before the pains began she had a large amount of fluid gush from her vagina. The pains are cramping type pains and are occuring five minutes apart, lasting about one minute each.

# ATV

## Bite or Sting

The patient has been bitten or stung by an insect and is having a localized reaction. Wash the area with antiseptic solution, remove the black spot if possible, and transport the patient to a medical facility. Be alert for changes in the patient's condition if the reaction becomes systemic.

## Which Protocol?

You arrive on the scene and find a woman in need of assistance. Your patient is a 55-year-old female who was working in her garden when she felt a sting on the back of her left arm. She is conscious, alert, and oriented times three in no apparent distress. She has no significant medical history, takes no medications, and has no known allergies. On the back of her left arm you note a bright red area approximately five inches in diameter with a small white area in the middle of the red area and a black spec in the middle of the white spot.

**All Terrain Vehicle:** Vehicles such as dirt bikes, three-wheelers, and four-wheelers designed for off-road use.

## Heat Exhaustion

The patient has a dimished level of consciousness due to a high core body temperature, yet her body is attempting to correct itself by perfuse sweating to lower her temperature. Place her in a cool ambulance, adminster oxygen, and transport to an emergency room.

## AVPU

Acronyms

**AVPU:** Mnemonic used to describe four levels of consciousness in order of importance: Alert, Verbal, Pain, Unresponsive

**Which Protocol?**

You respond to the scene of a road race for a female runner down. You arrive on scene and find a twenty-year-old female, conscious, breathing at a rate of 22 breaths-per-minute with a weak, thready pulse. Her skin is hot to the touch, and she is sweaty.

## Heat Stroke

This patient's sweating mechanism has been disrupted, causing her core body temperature to rise dramatically. Place the patient in a cool ambulance, administer oxygen, cover her head with a cool, wet towel, and transport priority to an emergency room.

# BLS

Acronyms

**Basic Life Support:** Protocols developed by the AHA to treat various cardiac conditions by an EMT-B, including CPR and AED.

**Which Protocol?**

You respond to the scene of a road race for a female runner down. You arrive on scene and find a twenty-year-old female, semi-conscious, breathing at a rate of 22 breaths-per-minute with a weak, thready pulse. Her skin is very hot to the touch, and there is no evidence of perspiration.

## Carbon Monoxide Poisoning

Administer oxygen at 15 liters per minute via non-rebreather mask and transport priority, preferably to a facility capable of treating carbon monoxide poisoning in a hyperbaric chamber.

## BP

**Blood pressure:** Pressure measured in millimeters of mercury of the blood flow through the arteries. Systolic blood pressure is the pressure in the arteries during ventricular contraction and diastolic blood pressure is the pressure in the arteries during ventricular relaxation.

**Which Protocol?**

You arrive on scene of an unkown type medical call and police lead you to a subject who is seated in his car, which is parked in his garage. The officer tells you that when they arrived the garage door was closed and the car was running. Police have shut the engine off and left the doors open. You enter the garage and observe a male seated behind the wheel of a car. He is unconscious and not responding to any stimuli. He is cyanotic, with slow shallow respirations and a weak, thready pulse.

## Hypoglycemia

IDDM stands for Insulin Dependent Diabetes Mellitus. This patient will respond almost immediately to the administration of oral glucose.

## BPM

Acronyms

**Beats per minute:** The number of times a pulse is felt in one minute.

**Which Protocol?**

You arrive at the scene of a call for medical aid. You find a male, aged 20, lying on his back. He is semi-conscious, but not alert. He is pale and diaphorretic. His pulse, blood pressure and respirations are normal and he has a medic-alert bracelet on his right wrist that says "IDDM."

# BSI

## Cardiac and Respiratory Arrest

Treatment for this patient will include CPR and application of the AED (Automated External Defibrillator). If the AED advises countershock, follow the prompts on the AED and defibrillate accordingly if indicated.

**Body Substance Isolation:** Those PPE measures (Personal Proctective Equipment measures) that protect the body from bloodborne and airborne pathogens; i.e. gloves, masks, eyewear, etc.

**Which Protocol?**

You arrive on the scene of a man down. He is unconscious and non-responsive, with no spontaneous respirations and no pulse.

## Chest Pain

Even in the absence of other possible cardiac symptoms, the protocols require intervention as though it may be a cardiac event. Lay the patient on the stretcher in a semi-Fowler position, apply the AED (Automated External Defibrillator), administer aspirin and oxygen per the local protocols, and transport priority.

# BVM

Acronyms

**Bag Valve Mask:** A device used to artificially ventilate a patient who is not breathing that consists of a pliable bag and a mask that fits over the patient's nose and mouth.

**Which Protocol?**

You arrive at the scene of an unknown type of medical emergency. You find a 44-year-old female patient sitting in her living room. She is guarding her left chest with her right hand. She is conscious, alert, and oriented times three. She states that the pain is 4 out of 10, non-radiating, and dull. She has no medical history, no allergies, and no prescriptions.

## Difficulty Breathing

The patient is obviously in respiratory distress and is anoxic, as indicated by his low oxygen saturation level. Administer oxygen 10 to 15 liters per minute by non-rebreather mask and transport priority.

# CHEMTREC

**Chemical Transportation Emergency Center:** A center for information on chemical accidents and spills that is provided by the chemical manufacturing industry and is available seven days a week, 24 hours a day.

**Which Protocol?**

You arrive at a residence to find a 60-year-old male seated at the kitchen table, hunched forward. His color is bluish and he is sweaty and cool to the touch. His respiratory rate is 22 and his SpO2 is 86%.

## Initial Assessment - ABC

In this situation, you must secure a patent airway. The correct sequence of treatment would be to take manual stablization of the patient's head and log roll him onto his back. Once on his back, perform a modified jaw thrust and ascertain whether or not he is breathing. If not, ventilate with two quick breaths and then check for a carotid pulse. If there is no pulse, begin CPR.

## CHF

**Congestive Heart Failure:** A cardiac condition where the heart fails to completely pump blood causing fluid to back up into the lungs (pulmonary edema).

**Which Protocol?**

You arrive on the scene of a motorcycle accident. The police have secured the scene, and you see a man lying prone on the ground in a puddle of blood. You are wearing suitable protective equipment. Which part of the assessment process is next, and which mnemonic are you going to use to help you ascertain an objective measurement of his complaint?

## Focused History and Physical Exam: Medical - SAMPLE

You have already completed the OPQRST portion of the survey and now you want her to again give you **S**igns and Symptoms, **A**llergies to Medications, **M**edications she is on, **P**ast Medical History, **L**ast Oral Intake and **E**vents leading up to this occurance. These questions are designed to help you narrow down the patient's condition so that you can present your findings to the emergency room physician or triage nurse.

## CISD

**Critical Incident Stress Debriefing:** A formal group or individual counseling session following a stressful incident such as a mass casualty incident or the death of a child.

**Which Protocol?**

You arrive at an office building for an unknown type medical call. The patient is sobbing quietly, holding her head in her hands. She appears to be in distress and somewhat reluctant to answer your questions. She says she is having the worst headache of her life, and that the pain came upon her suddenly as she was looking at her computer screen constructing a spreadsheet. She says that the pain goes from her temples upward and then to the back of her head. It is a ten out of ten, and she has never experienced anything like it before. Which part of the assessment process is next, and which mnemonic are you going to use to help you ascertain an objective measurement of her complaint?

## Focused History and Physical Exam: Trauma – DCAP-BTLS

In examining the lower leg you want to note: Is there any **D**eformity, **C**ontusion, **A**brasion, **P**uncture, **B**urn, **T**enderness, **L**aceration, or **S**welling?



$CO_2$

**Carbon Dioxide:** The gas given off by the cells as a by-product of cellular metabolism.

**Which Protocol?**

You respond to the front of the local library for a woman who has fallen. She is complaining of pain to her right lower leg, but otherwise appears uninjured. Which part of the assessment process is next, and which mnemonic are you going to use to help you ascertain an objective measurement of her complaint?

## Focused History and Physical Exam: Medical - OPQRST

When did the pain begin? (**O**nset). Did any special activity cause it to occur? (**P**rovacation). Can you describe the pain? (**Q**uality). Does the pain move anywhere else? (**R**adiation). Can you describe the level of pain on a scale from one to ten, ten being the worst? (**S**everity). How long have you had the pain and have you ever felt anything like it before? (**T**ime).



## COPD

**Chronic Obstructive Pulmonary Disease:** Mainly two diseases, emphysema and chronic bronchitis, where the lung tissue becomes obstructed by the disease and inhibits the oxygen/carbon dioxide exchange.

**Which Protocol?**

You are dispatched to a residence for a patient with abdominal pains. You arrive on scene and the patient is seated on the couch. He is conscious, alert and oriented times three, and is guarding his right abdomen with his left arm, complaining of pain. Which part of the assessment process is next, and which mnemonic are you going to use to help you ascertain an objective measurement of his complaint?

## Hypothermia (Second stage)

In addition to the injuries you may find in the ongoing assessment, your patient is also suffering from second stage hypothermia and needs to be gradually warmed, in addition to having any injuries you may find treated. The absence of shivering means that he has passed through first stage hypothermia and has entered second stage.



# CPR

**Cardio Pulmonary Resuscitation:** Treatment of a patient with no pulse or respiration, which consists of artificial ventilation and chest compressions.

**Which Protocol?**

You arrive at a motor vehicle accident on a cold, snowy night. The road is lightly traveled, it is early in the morning and the vehicle has struck a tree. Your patient is semi-conscious, incoherent, and tachypneic with a weak thready pulse. You smell alcoholic beverages in his exhaled breath. His skin is cold and dry to the touch, but he is not shivering.

# CSF

## Allergic Reaction

If allowed by your protocols, immediately administer .3mg of 1:1000 Epinephrine by auto-injector, administer oxygen 10-15 liters per minute by non-rebreather mask and transport priority. Her signs and syptoms are classic anaphylaxis (allergic reaction) and seafood and shellfish are common food allergens.

**Cerebral Spinal Fluid:** Fluid from the skull or spinal column. When CSF is seen in the ears, nose, or mouth as a result of trauma it is indicative of serious internal injury to the brain.

**Which Protocol?**

You respond to a restaurant for a female in distress. The patient has a hand to her throat and appears to be having difficulty breathing; her lips are swollen and she has a rash all over her face. Her companion is upset and has no knowledge of her medical history. He states that she ate a shrimp from the shrimp cocktail when the symptoms began. The police officer hands you an Epi-Pen from the patient's handbag.

# CVA

## Sudden Death

You may be tempted to begin CPR with this patient, but his signs and symptoms indicate that biological (irreversible) death has occurred. No further medical intervention is necessary. Document all of the applicable information and turn the matter over to the police.

**Cerebral Vascular Accident:** A blood clot or bleeding inside the brain causing death of brain tissue, also known as a stroke.

**Which Protocol?**

You are dispatched to meet the police at a residence. You enter the dwelling and you find a male, lying supine, his eyes open, his color cyanotic. You attempt to perform the airway maneuver and you find that his jaw is rigid and will not open. He has no respirations or pulse. His skin is cold to the touch and his wrist and elbow are also rigid. As you look at his chest, you notice that the anterior is pale and bluish, but the posterior aspect is blackish.

# DCAP-BTLS

## Cardiopulmonary Resuscitation

Place the patient on the floor or on a backboard, open his airway with a head-tilt, chin lift, and ventilate him twice. If you get chest rise and air exchange, check for a carotid pulse. If it is absent, begin chest compressions. Apply the AED (Automatic External Defibrillator) and shock if instructed. Continue CPR and transport.

**DCAP-BTLS:** Another mnemonic for physical examination, but more comprehensive than DOTS; Deformities, Contusions (bruises), Abrasions, Punctures, Burns, Tenderness, Lacerations, and Swelling

**Which Protocol?**

You are dispatched for a medical aid. You arrive on the scene to find a 70-year-old male sitting at the kitchen table, clutching his chest. He suddenly goes unconscious and his head hits the table. He now has no pulse, no respirations, and no blood pressure.

# DDT

## Chest Pain

This patient has all the classic symptoms of a heart attack. Administer oxygen 10-15 liters-per-minute via non-rebreather mask, administer 325 mg of aspirin if allowed by protocol, and ask if the patient takes nitrogylcerin. Apply the AED (Automatic External Defibrillator) and transport priority.

**Which Protocol?**

You arrive at the police station to find a male sitting in the lobby. He is pale and sweating heavily with his right hand over his middle chest. He appears to be having mild difficulty breathing and his vital signs are BP 100/60, respirations 18 and pulse 120. He is conscious, alert, oriented times 3, and states that it feels like there is an elephant sitting on his chest.

**Dichloro Diphenyl Trichlorethane:** A highly-toxic insecticide, which is currently banned.

## Load and Go Transport

This patient presents multiple symptoms that indicate conditions that can only be treated in a hospital. After the rapid assessment, he should be packaged and transported priority.

# DECON

**Decontamination of Hazardous Materials:** If either a patient or a provider is contaminated by hazardous materials on a scene, she must be decontaminated, or deconned, on the scene.

**Which Protocol?**

You arrive at a motor vehicle accident. Your patient was riding a bicycle when he was struck by a car. He is unconscious and non-responsive to painful stimuli. His breathing is irregular, his blood pressure is 100 by palpation, and his pulse is 120.

# DNR

## Scene Safety

This type of call is an example of an unsafe condition; if you proceed it will expose you and your crew to a dangerous situation for which you are not equipped to defend against. Withdraw and wait for the police to secure the scene.

**Do Not Resuscitate:** An advanced directive by a terminally ill patient advising that in the event of cardiac or pulmonary arrest he is not to be revived.

**Which Protocol?**

You arrive at a call to assist the police. As you pull up to the residence, you notice a female lying prone in front of the residence and you hear gunshots coming from the residence.

## Difficulty Breathing

She is breathing and has a pulse, so her ABC's are OK. There is no sign of gross hemorrhage, but her oxygen saturation is low. Administer oxygen via non-rebreather at 10-15 liters-per-minute and prepare to transport.

Acronyms

## DOT

**Department of Transportation:** The federal agency which promulgated rules and protocols for EMS in response to the mandates of the National Highway Safety Act of 1966.

**Which Protocol?**

You are dispatched for an unkown type rescue. You enter a bedroom and see a sixty-year-old female sitting on the edge of the bed hunched forward. She is gasping for air, her blood pressure is 180/60, her pulse is 100, and her pulse oximetry saturation is 84%.

## Foreign Body Airway Obstruction

You must clear the airway before ventilating. You should place the child on his back, provide five quick thrusts to his abdomen, check to see if anything is now in the airway, and attempt to re-ventilate.

---

## DOTS

Acronyms

**DOTS:** Mnemonic used to recall things to look for when examining a patient: Deformities, Open injuries, Tenderness, Swelling

**Which Protocol?**

You respond to a residence for a child not breathing. You arrive on the scene and the mother thrusts her four year old son into your arms. He is unconscious, cyanotic, and non-responsive. You attempt to ventilate with a pocket mask, but you feel resistance and you get no chest rise or air exchange.

# EMS

## Airway

This patient will probably respond immediately to having his airway opened with a head-tilt, chin lift, or jaw thrust maneuver.

**Emergency Medical Services:** System of providing emergency pre-hospital care to the population inlcuding assessment, treatment of life threatening conditions, and transport to a medical facility.

**Which Protocol?**

You respond to a nursing home for medical transport. You arrive in the patient's room and he is lying on his back, unconscious and non-responsive, gasping for air.

## Seizure

The patient is probably suffering from a febrile seizure caused by his high temperature. Treatment would include oxygen, airway management, and transport. Consider applying a cool towel to the head to lower the patient's temperature.

**Emergency Medical Technician, Basic:** The licensing level which enables provider to perform Basic Life Support protocols such as drug administration, patient assessment, and transport.

**Which Protocol?**

You arrive on the scene of an unknown type rescue to find a 4-year-old male shaking uncontrolably, eyes rolled back into head, BP 100/60, pulse 80, respirations undetermined. Rectal temperature is 105 degrees.

If the patient exhibits signs and symptoms of stroke, including high blood pressure, facial droop and muscle weakness on one side, administer oxygen at a rate of 10-15 liters per minute by non-rebreather mask and transport priority to a hospital emergency room.

**Emergency Medical Technician, Intermediate:** The licensing level which enables the provider to perform some advanced life support protocols such as endotracheal intubation, IV administration, and manual cardio-version.

**STROKE**

**Treatment Modalities**

# EMT-P

As the body responds to a serious injury, the loss of blood becomes more problematic. If the bleeding has been controlled, keep the patient warm by applying blankets and elevate the feet to a point higher than the head (Trendelenburg position). Monitor the patient's vital signs closely and, if protocols allow, consider application of Pneumatic Anti Shock Garment.

**Emergency Medical Technician, Paramedic:** The licensing level which enables provider to perform most advanced life support protocols including some surgical interventions such as cricothoratomy and pleural decompression.

**SHOCK**

**Treatment Modalities**

# FBAO

In the event of severe bleeding, the first intervention is to apply direct pressure with a sterile dressing. If this is not successful in controlling the bleeding, apply pressure on an artery pressure point leading to the wound. This may slow the flow of blood enough to allow the bleeding to clot. If neither of these measures is effective, then a tourniquet of a broad strip of cloth should be placed as close to the wound as is possible and tightened until the bleeding stops. Medical control should be notified, and the time the tourniquet is applied should be noted.

**Foreign Body Airway Obstruction:** Condition where an object, usually food, blocks the airway and requires a combination of abdominal thrusts and back blows to clear the obstruction.

## SEVERE BLEEDING

Treatment Modalities

Usually grand mal seizures last one to two minutes and are then followed by a period of unconsciousness or semi-consciousness. If the seizure is still active, place a bite stick between the patient's teeth to prevent clamping down on his/her tongue and hold the head to keep the airway open. Once the seizure has stopped, transport the patient priority to an emergency room.

# FCC

**Federal Communication Commission:** The federal agency responsible for licensing and assigning communications frequencies. FCC Part 95 is the standard which assigns Public Safety Radio frequencies.

## SEIZURES

Treatment Modalities

This type of call is complicated since a number of factors need to be addressed. The patient's medical condition is always the primary concern and a gentle, confident approach is needed. If possible, the primary provider should be of the same gender as the patient. Clothing that has to removed or cut should be kept in a plastic bag for evidence. Physical examination of the patient should be limited to those things that are acute, since the patient will be sensitive to touch and visualization of genitals. This examination is best done in the emergency room, however severe bleeding and wound management must be done as soon as possible in the field.

## FR

**First Responder:** The licensing level which allows non-medical public safety officials such as police officer and firefighters to perform basic first aid and preliminary life support measures such as cardio pulmonary resuscitation and automatic external defibrillation.

## RAPE AND SEXUAL ASSAULT

**Treatment Modalities**

**Acronyms**

# HAZMAT

If a patient has ingested a non-caustic, non-petroleum poison, contact medical control for possible administration of syrup of ipecac, which will cause vomiting within approximately 15 minutes. When the patient vomits, have him on his side and protect the airway, and have suctioning equipment ready. In the event of caustics and petroleum products, transport priority and contact medical control for possible administration of activated charcoal solution to slow the absorption of the toxin into the blood stream.

**Hazardous Materials:** Any substance which may cause illness or death when exposed to a human being.

## POISONING

Treatment Modalities

A patient who is not breathing should immediately be checked for an open airway. Once the airway is opened by either the head-tilt, chin lift method or by the modified jaw thrust, two breaths should be administered either by bag valve mask or pocket mask. Respirations should be continued at a rate of one each five seconds.

## HBV

**Hepatitis B Virus:** A bloodborne pathogen which causes liver damage.

**PATIENT NOT BREATHING**

**Treatment Modalities**

In the case of fractures of the torso (ribs, sternum, clavicle, scapula, etc.) packing the injured area with a soft object and securing it in place to prevent motion is often the best emergency treatment.

# HEPA

## Acronyms

**High Efficiency Particulate Air:** A type of mask used to filter airborne particulates which cause disease, such as tubercolis-infected saliva droplets.

## OTHER FRACTURE

Treatment Modalities

Open wounds should be treated in the field prior to transport or during transport if the patient is a load and go. Irrigate the wounds with sterile water to remove foreign material. Place a sterile dressing on the wound and secure it with bandaging material. Remember that the emergency room staff is going to want to visualize the wound, so do not put on too much bandaging material.

## HIV

**Human Immunodeficiency Virus:** The virus that causes AIDS. This pathogen is passed from one infected person to another by blood, semen, vaginal, or cervical secretions.

**OPEN WOUNDS**

Treatment Modalities

If a patient is being ventilated by another person and also has no pulse, then chest compressions should begin immediately at a rate of 60 per minute. On an adult, measure two finger widths from the tip of the sternum and place the other palm on the sternum. Place the other hand on top and begin to compress one and a half to two inches.

# IC

**Incident Commander:** The person in charge of any event in which an ICS (Incident Command System) is established. He or she will direct three people or groups, who in turn will each direct three people or groups.

**NO PULSE**

**Treatment Modalities**

# ICS

After delivery, use care in handling the baby as he will be slippery. Suction the baby's nose and mouth of fluid, and if the baby does not start to breath spontaneously, rub his back vigorously. After one minute, note the baby's appearance, pulse, grimace, activity, and respiration (APGAR score). If respiration is absent, begin artificial ventilation and if there is no pulse, begin CPR.

**Incident Command System:** A command system based upon the U.S. military command structure, which basically states that one person can be in direct command of no more than three functions.

# NEONATE POST-PARTUM CARE

Treatment Modalities

# IDDM

After the umbilical cord is cut, prepare for the delivery of the placenta. Place the placenta in a clean basin. After delivery of the placenta, place two sanitary napkins over the mother's vagina and have her lower her legs and place them together. Massage her uterus to facilitate the stoppage of bleeding and continue transporting to a maternity facility.

**Insulin Dependent Diabetes Mellitus:** A disease of the endocrine system where the body no longer produces insulin, leading to high sugar levels in the blood. Treatment consists of injecting synthetic insulin to maintain steady sugar levels.

## MATERNAL POST-PARTUM CARE

Treatment Modalities

Acronyms

# LLQ

The goal in management of long bone fractures is to immobilize the broken bone ends and the adjacent joints. This is accomplished by applying the proper splint and securing it to prevent motion of the affected limb.

**Left Lower Quadrant:** The quarter of the abdomen determined by the left side of the patient and below the navel.

## LONG BONE FRACTURES

Treatment Modalities

# LPM

Remove the patient's wet clothing and perform a complete assessment of his condition. Slowly warm the patient by placing him in a warm truck and covering him with warm blankets. Heat packs or heated IV bags may be placed in the groin and armpits to expedite the warming process.

**Liters Per Minute:** A unit of volume measurement in delivery of oxygen gas to a patient.

**HYPOTHERMIA**

**Treatment Modalities**

Place the patient in a cool spot. If the patient is perspiring, place a cool towel on the head and help her drink an electrolyte solution such as Gatorade, if available, or water. If the patient is hot and dry, expedite transport and use air conditioning and wet sheets to lower her temperature. Cold packs in the groin and armpits may also help lower core temperature.

# LUQ

**Left Upper Quadrant:** The quarter of the abdomen determined by the left side of the patient and above the navel.

**HYPERTHERMIA**

**Treatment Modalities**

If a wound is present, treat according to burn or wound protocols. The potential for cardiac dysrhythmia as a result of an electrical shock is of particular concern. If the shock passed through the chest area, it is prudent to apply the AED (Automatic External Defibrillator) pads in preparation for having to analyze a dysrthymia and possible counter shock.

## LZ

**Landing Zone:** A clear space set up to receive helicopters for bringing in supplies and extricating patients from a situation.

Crew safety is paramount. If the patient is unconscious, then treat as a poisoning or overdose. If the patient is conscious, then use a calm voice to get the patient to do what you need him to do. If he becomes violent or out of control, then contact medical control for permission to restrain. Always have a sufficient number of personnel on hand to apply restraints and restrain the patient to a backboard, supine with one hand at his side and the other above his head. Be sure to use sufficient straps to hold the patient down. Constantly monitor the patient's airway and pulse and transport priority.



## MCI

**Mass Casualty Incident:** Defined as having one more patient than the responding unit can handle, necessitating the dispatching of additional units. An MCI usually requires the implementation of the ICS (Incident Command System).

## DRUG AND ALCOHOL ABUSE

### Treatment Modalities

If a patient is conscious and alert and complaining of difficulty breathing, assess the percentage of oxygen saturation with a pulse oximeter and record this for the emergency room. If the difficulty breathing is severe and the pulse oximeter reading is less than 90%, immediately administer oxygen at a rate of 10-15 liters-per-minute via a non-rebreather mask. If the difficulty is moderate and the pulse oximeter is greater than 90%, consider administering oxygen using a nasal cannula at rate of two to six liters per minute.



## MSDS

**Manufacturer's Safety Data Sheet:** Printout provided with all hazardous materials, including first aid information, hazard information, fire suppression information, and exposure limits.

DIFFICULTY BREATHING

Treatment Modalities

If you suspect hypoglycemia, check the blood sugar with the glucometer. If the patient is conscious, obtain medical control permission to administer glucose gel by squirting it along his gums. If the patient is unconscious, some systems may allow the injection of glucagon, a hormone which releases sugar stored in the liver.

## NC

**Nasal Cannula:** An oxygen delivery device placed in a patient's nostrils which will deliver between 20 to 40% oxygen at a liter flow rate of 2 to 6 liters per minute.

## DIABETIC EMERGENCIES

Treatment Modalities

Emergency childbirth is a natural process. If delivery is imminent, stop the vehicle and place the mother in a semi-Fowler position with her legs elevated. As the contractions begin, encourage the mother to push and place one hand below the vagina to support the head as it is delivered and gently guide the head out with the other hand to prevent an explosive delivery. Once the head is out, the baby will rotate and the remainder of the delivery is usually quick.

# NFPA

**National Fire Protection Association:** A private group responsible for establishing standards for fire protection and fire suppression. It has also established some standards for fire-service-based EMS.

CHILDBIRTH

Treatment Modalities

Child abuse is usually secondary to another condition, such as broken bones and wounds. All medical conditions must be cared for first. If the provider suspects child abuse, it is his responsibility to notify the agency responsible for investigating child abuse allegations. The report to the agency must be factual and complete, covering all aspects of the scene examination and patient care.

## 911

Acronyms

**911:** Universal emergency reporting telephone number. Dialing this number connects the caller to a dispatch center that will summon EMS and other public safety officials to any emergency. Enhanced 911 systems provide the location of the caller to the dispatcher.

## CHILD ABUSE

**Treatment Modalities**

Place the patient in a comfortable position, usually sitting up at a forty five degree angle. If permitted by local protocol, administer oxygen via non-rebreather mask at 10-15 liters per minute, administer 325 mg aspirin orally and have the patient chew it, then transport the patient priority to an emergency room. While en route place the AED (Automatic External Defibrillator) pads on the patient. If the patient has nitroglycerine, contact medical control for permission to assist the patient in taking it as directed.

## N95

**N95:** A HEPA Mask that filters out 95% of airbone particulates.

CHEST PAIN

Treatment Modalities

Burns are treated as wounds. It is important to note as part of the assessment the amount of body surface affected and the degree of the burns: superficial, partial thickness, and full thickness. Cooling of the burn with sterile water is helpful in pain management. Also, the airway must constantly be checked since airway compromise from swelling is always a concern if heat has been inhaled.

## NRB

**Non Rebreather Mask:** An oxygen delivery device placed over a patient's nose and mouth that delivers 80 to 100% oxygen at a liter flow rate of 10 to 15 liters per minute.

**BURNS**

**Treatment Modalities**

In addition to providing basic life support, remove the stinger if still in the wound and treat the wound. Try to identify the object that bit or stung the patient and transport priority to an emergency room.

**National Registry of Emergency Medical Technicians:** Provides national licensing exams and registration for EMTs and paramedics.

BITES AND STINGS

Treatment Modalities

The safety of the crew is paramount in dealing with a patient who may be mentally ill. Often, all that is needed to get the patient to obey your directions is having a calm approach and showing that you have empathy for the patient and can identify with his problem. In the event that a patient is violent and out of control, contact medical control to request permission to restrain. Always have a sufficient number of personnel on hand to apply restraints and restrain the patient to a backboard, supine with one hand at his side and the other above his head and sufficient straps to hold the patient down. Constantly monitor the patient's airway and pulse and transport priority, minimizing the use of the siren.

## OB-GYN

**Acronyms**

**Obstetrics and Gynecology:** Medical specialty comprising the study and treatment of childbearing and female reproductive systems.

**BEHAVIOR EMERGENCIES**

**Treatment Modalities**

Administer oxygen via non-rebreather at 10-15 liters-per-minute. If permitted by local protocols, check blood glucose with a glucometer. If the reading is less than 60, contact medical control for permission to treat for low blood sugar. Transport priority to an emergency room and perform a complete assessment en route.

## OPQRST

**OPQRST:** Mnemonic used to remember questions asked regarding an abnormal condition such as pain. It stands for: Onset, Provocation, Quality, Region, Radiation, Relief, Severity, Time

ALTERED MENTAL STATUS

Treatment Modalities

# OSHA

If a patient exhibits difficulty breathing and hives secondary to a possible allergic reaction, contact medical control for permission to administer an auto injector of epinephrine into the thigh muscle. First prep the site with an alcohol wipe. Then remove the safety cap from the injector, make sure that the needle end is on the thigh, and push.

**Occupational Safety and Health Administration:** A division of the Department of Labor that promulgates rules for worker safety and investigates accidents in the workplace.

## ALLERGIC REACTIONS

Treatment Modalities

If you cannot ventilate a patient and feel an obstruction in the airway, reposition the airway and try again. If the airway is still obstructed, straddle the patient's legs and locate the inferior end of the sternum (xiphoid process) and place two hands on the stomach below this point and push in and up five times. Open the mouth and check for a foreign object with your fingers. If an object is located, remove it and retry ventilation. If nothing is found, repeat the abdominal compressions until successful or until instructed to cease by medical control.

## $O_2$

**$O_2$:** The chemical symbol for oxygen, which is an element necessary for a human being to metabolize fuel for life. Withdrawal of oxygen to the brain will result in death in approximately five minutes under normal circumstances.

## AIRWAY OBSTRUCTION

Treatment Modalities

# PAD

Perform a complete medical assessment and transport the patient to an emergency room. Common causes of abdominal pain include appendicitis, gastroenteritis, gynecological problems, and others. If as you are palpating the abdomen you feel a pulsating mass, this is a possible abdominal aortic aneurysm and transport should be expedited.

**Public Access Defibrillation:** AEDs which are available for use in public venues such as shopping malls, sport arenas, airports, and other large gathering areas.

## ABDOMINAL PAIN

Treatment Modalities

These combination dressing and bandage packages are not used often, but are indespensible in a major wound situation. There should be a minimum of two in the truck and one in the trauma bag.



## PAT

**Pediatric Assessment Triangle:** Tool for assessing the pediatric patient; Appearance (AVPU scale), Breathing (airway, breathing effort, and head/torso color), and Circulation (pulse rate/strength, extremity color, capillary refill, and blood pressure).

## TRAUMA DRESSINGS

Truck Check Items

# PCR

Towels are necessary for cleaning and for absorbing various fluids. A minimum of six cloth towels should be carried on the truck, along with a roll of paper towels.

**Prehospital Care Report:** Form on which an EMS encounter with a patient is documented.

**TOWELS**

**Truck Check Items**

Acronyms

# PE

An electronic device used to determine a patient's core body temperature. There should be one on the truck or in the medical bag.

**Physical Exam:** The visual examination of a patient for signs and symptoms of illness or injury.

## THERMOMETER

Truck Check Items

# PPE

Adhesive tape is used to secure sterile dressings if more applicable than using adhering bandages. It is also used to tape the end of the self adhering bandage to make it more secure. There should be a large number of surgical quality tape rolls in various widths (1 inch, 2 inch and 3 inch) in both the truck and trauma bag.

**Personal Protective Equipment:** All of those items used by EMS personnel to protect themselves from the hazards of emergency medicine, including but not limited to disposable gloves, eye protection, gowns, and HEPA and N95 masks.

**TAPE**

**Truck Check Items**

Acronyms

# PSI

A device used for listening to various sounds in the body as part of patient assessment. There should be one in the kit that is carried and one in the truck.

**Pounds per Square Inch:** A unit of pressure measurement used to determine how much oxygen or other compressed gas remains in a cylinder.

# STETHOSCOPE

Truck Check Items

# PTO

These are dressings used to control bleeding. There should be a large number of these of in various sizes (2x2 inches, 4x4 inches, 5x9 inches ) in the truck and in the trauma bag.

**Power Take Off:** Means of powering auxiliary units of machinery from a main power source, e.g. using the engine of a farm tractor to run the operation of a towed hay baler.

Truck Check Items

**STERILE DRESSINGS**

These are rigid or semi-rigid boards or other devices that are used to immobilize a suspected fracture or sprain. There should be at least two short rigid splints and two long rigid splints on the truck, in addition to a full set of inflatable or velcro vinyl splints. The full set includes splints for foot and ankle, half leg, full leg, hand and wrist, half arm, and full arm.

# PTSD

**Post Traumatic Stress Disorder:** A physical and psychological response to stressful situations. The signs and symptoms of PTSD may include loss of appetite, anger, depression, loss of sexual interest, irritability, difficulty sleeping, and nightmares.

**SPLINTS**

**Truck Check Items**

Sheets are placed on the stretcher to help maintain a clean environment for treating and transporting patients. A minimum of two spare sheets and two spare pillow cases should be carried on the truck.

# RLQ

**Right Lower Quadrant:** The quarter of the abdomen determined by the right side of the patient and below the navel.

**SHEETS**

Truck Check Items

# RUQ

Containers which allow for the safe collection of used sharp objects such as needles and glass tubes. There should be one in the kit that is carried and one in the truck.

**Right Upper Quadrant:** The quarter of the abdomen determined by the right side of the patient and above the navel.

## SHARPS CONTAINER

Truck Check Items

# SAMPLE

Self adhering bandages are used to secure sterile dressings to the patient's wounds. There should be a large number of these in various widths (2 inch, 3 inch, and 4 inch) in the truck and in the trauma bag.

**SAMPLE:** Mnemonic used to remember questions asked during a patient exam; Signs and symptoms, Allergies, Medications, Past history, Last oral intake, and Events leading up to current problem

**SELF ADHERING BANDAGES**

Truck Check Items

# SCBA

A two-way radio is necessary for communication with the dispatcher and the receiving hospitals. The truck radio and all communication equipment should be checked for proper operations at the beginning of each shift.

**Self-Contained Breathing Apparatus:** A portable air supply used to enter a hazardous atmosphere.

## RADIO

Truck Check Items

# SIDS

An electronic instrument that measures the level of oxygen in the hemoglobin as a function of the respiration and circulation. There should be one in the truck.

**Sudden Infant Death Syndrome:** A condition where an infant or toddler dies suddenly with no discernible cause.

PULSE OXIMETER

Truck Check Items

# SSSSS

The portable suction unit is used to remove fluids form a patient's airway to facilitate breathing and ventilation. The portable suction unit should be carried in the airway or medical bag and should be checked for proper operation at the beginning of each shift.

**SSSSS:** Five steps to be taken by a first responder arriving at the scene of an MCI (Mass Casualty Incident) or WMD (Weapons of Mass Destruction) incident: Self (The safety of the responder is a first priority.), Size up (What are we dealing with? How many victims are there? What type and number of resources will be needed?), Send info (Communicate with your communications center and advise them of what you've found up to that point.), Set up medical group (EMS will be responsible for triage, treatment, and transport of the injured.), Stabilize (Attempt to gain control of the situation.)

## PORTABLE SUCTION UNIT

**Truck Check Items**

# START

All portable oxygen cylinders should have a minimum of 500 pounds-per-square-inch and should be replaced if they contain less. There should also be one spare full cylinder for each portable oxygen device in use.

**Simple Triage and Rapid Transport:** System of triage at a mass-casualty incident. Each patient is assigned a color code based on the seriousness of their injuries: red for critical; yellow for serious; green for minor; and black for fatal injuries.

# PORTABLE OXYGEN

Truck Check Items

# TB

Non-permeable material to cover wounds in the chest and neck and prevent air leakage. There should be a minimum of two in the truck and two in the trauma bag.

**Tuberculosis:** A lung disease caused by airborne particulates contaminated with the tuberculin bacteria.

# OCCLUSIVE DRESSINGS

Truck Check Items

There should be one mask for each oxygen tank in use, as well as one spare for each. If there is a portable unit and a truck unit, there should be a total of four masks.

# V-FIB

**Ventricular Fibrillation:** A cardiac condition where the electrical activity of the heart is insufficient to provide enough ventricular contraction to produce a pulse and adequate circulation.

## NON-REBREATHER MASKS

Truck Check Items

Acronyms

# VS

Disposable items that make liquid medications such as epinephrine and albuterol into mists that can be inhaled into the lungs. If local protocols allow the administration of nebulized medications, there should be a minimum of two nebulizers on the truck.

**Vital Signs:** Measurements of body function such as blood pressure, respiratory rate, and pulse rate.

There should be one cannula for each oxygen tank in use, as well as one spare for each. If there is a portable unit and a truck unit, then there should be a total of four cannula.



# V-TACH

**Ventricular tachycardia:** Cardiac condition where the ventricles of the heart are beating too fast to produce a pulse and adequate circulation.

## NASAL CANNULA

Truck Check Items

# WMD

The main oxygen tank on the truck should have a minimum of 400 pounds-per-square-inch of oxygen and should be replaced if it contains less.

**Weapons of Mass Destruction:** Devices causing a large amount of destruction and injury. Examples of WMDs include radiological agents, chemical agents, biological agents and explosive agents.

**MAIN TRUCK OXYGEN**

Truck Check Items

The main stretcher is used to transport almost all patients and is mounted to the floor or the walls of the truck. It is adjustable and can be used in different configurations, such as Trendelenberg or semi-Fowler. The stretcher should be checked for proper operation in all positions and should be made up according to the protocols of the service with a minimum of two sheets, one blanket, one pillow, and one towel.

# ACTIVATED CHARCOAL

A fairly benign substance which absorbs toxins in the digestive tract and helps prevent them from entering the bloodstream.

MAIN STRETCHER

Truck Check Items

# ALBUTEROL

A KED or short spine board is a splinting device that is used where a long backboard cannot be utilized, such as inside a motor vehicle following a crash. There should be a minimum of one on the truck.

A drug that when given by nebulizer causes the airways in the lungs to dilate and reduces respiratory distress.

## KED OR SHORT SPINE BOARD

**Truck Check Items**

Head blocks are fastened to the backboard to secure the head and neck to the backboard. There should be a minimum of two sets of head blocks, one for each backboard carried on the truck, each with a set of two securing straps.

# ASPIRIN (ASA)

Pain reliever given for relief of chest pain. Aspirin also inhibits the clotting action of the blood platelets and may help relieve blockages in the coronary arteries during a heart attack.

## HEAD BLOCKS

Truck Check Items

An electronic device that measures the blood sugar level in a drop of blood. There should be one in either the truck or in the medical bag.

# EPINEPHRINE (EPI)

Synthetic adrenaline indicated for treatment of an allergic reaction.

## GLUCOMETER

Truck Check Items

# GLUCOSE

The truck should always have a minimum of half a tank of fuel. Many services require their units to be filled at the end of each shift.

Concentrated sugar in gel form given to patients with low blood sugar.

**FUEL**

**Truck Check Items**

# IPECAC

These bandages are used to support injured joints, especially sprained ankles. They come in a variety of widths such as 2 inch, 3 inch, 4 inch, and 5 inch. At least one of each width should be carried in the truck and in the trauma bag.

An emetic that induces vomiting and may be indicated for the treatment of poisoning and/or drug overdose.

**ELASTIC BANDAGES**

Truck Check Items

The following drugs should be carried on BLS units, subject to local protocols: albuterol (difficulty breathing), insta-glucose (low blood sugar), aspirin (chest pain), epinephrine (chest pain), nitroglycerine tablets or spray (chest pain), ipecac (poisoning and overdose), activated charcoal (poisoning and overdose), and ammonia capsules (loss of consciousness).

# NITROGLYCERIN (NTG)

A potent drug which causes arteries to dilate and reduces blood pressure while increasing blood flow to the heart.

**DRUGS**

Truck Check Items

These are necessary as part of each EMT's personal protective equipment to minimize the danger of bloodborne pathogens. There should be a box of each size carried on the truck. In addition, each crew person should have two sets on their person in the size that he or she uses.

# OXYGEN ($O_2$)

A compressed component of air that is used by cells to metabolize. When given medically at a higher percentage than the surrounding atmosphere, it often helps alleviate respiratory distress.

Truck Check Items

**DISPOSABLE GLOVES**

# ANTERIOR

Non-sterile cloth bandage materials that come in large triangle shapes and can be readily rolled or twisted into a long shape and used to secure a dressing on any part of the body. There should be a minimum of three in the truck and three in the trauma bag.

The front side of the body.

Truck Check Items

**CRAVATS**

# DISTAL

Disposable bags into which a patient may vomit. There should be two in the kit that is carried and a package of them in the truck.

Away from.

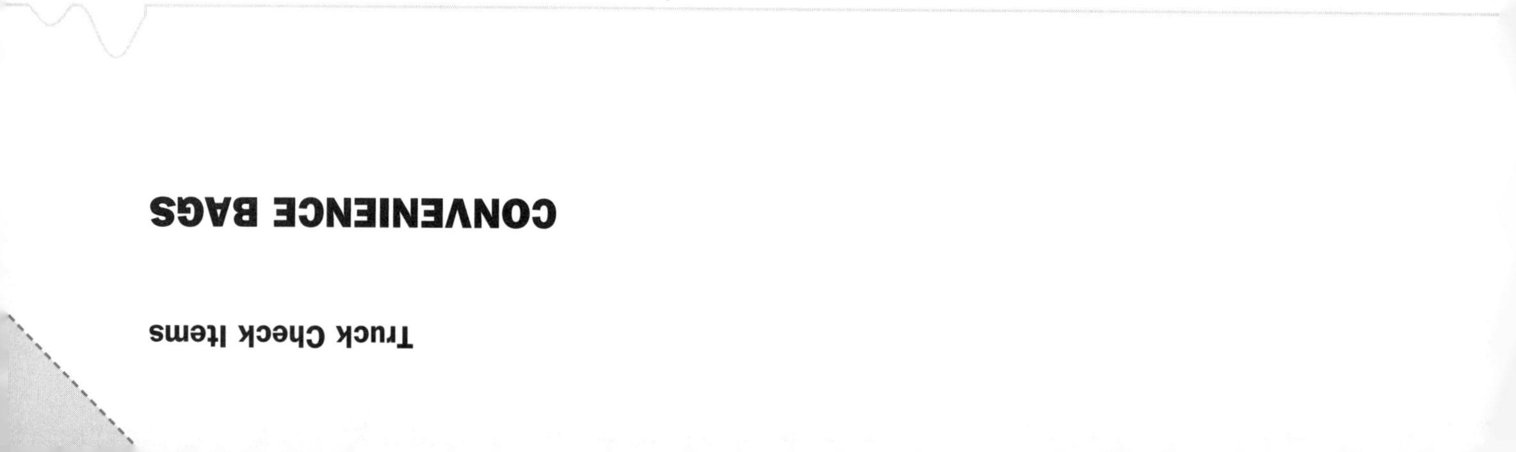

# INFERIOR

These are splinting devices which will help to maintain cervical stabilization in the event of suspected trauma. There should be a minimum of two of each adult size (tall, regular, short, and no-neck) and one of each pediatric size (regular, infant, and infant no-neck).

Below the horizontal midline.

**CERVICAL COLLARS**

**Truck Check Items**

# LATERAL

A device used for measuring blood pressure. There should be one in the kit that is carried and one in the truck.

Away from the vertical midline.

**BP CUFF**

**Truck Check Items**

# MEDIAL

Blankets are used to cover patients and are critical in cold temperatures to help the patient maintain warmth. A minimum of two spare blankets should be carried on the truck.

Towards the vertical middle or midline.

**BLANKETS**

**Truck Check Items**

Anatomy–Bones of the Skull

# PARIETAL

A disposable item used for artificial ventilation of a person who has stopped breathing. There should be one in the kit that is carried and one in the truck.

The bones which form the top and sides of the skull covering the brain.

**BAG VALVE MASK**

Truck Check Items

# POSTERIOR (DORSAL)

Backboards are essentially long splinting devices which help to immobilize the spinal column and minimize movement of the vertebral column and protect the spinal cord. There should be a minimum of two backboards carried on the truck. (They are also known as spineboards.)

The back side of the body.

**BACKBOARDS**

Truck Check Items

**Anatomy–Descriptions of the Body**

# PROXIMAL

These straps are used to secure a patient to a backboard. There should be a minimum of two sets of backboard straps, one for each backboard carried on the truck, each with a set of four securing straps.

Located next to or near.

## BACKBOARD STRAPS

Truck Check Items

# SUPERIOR

The AED (Automated External Defibrillator) is a device that will shock a heart that is fibrillating back into a normal sinus rhythm. The AED should be carried on the truck and brought along on any possible heart call for immediate emergency defibrillation. It should be checked for proper operation according to the manufacturer's recommendations at the start of every shift.

Above the horizontal midline.

**AED**

**Truck Check Items**

# MANDIBLE

An alcohol or other antiseptic-based cleaner and sanitizer to be used after patient contact, which helps to prevent the spread of bacteria and viruses.

The lower part of the front skull; the jawbone.

**WATERLESS HAND CLEANER**

Medical Equipment

# MASTOID

A pressure bandage applied tightly enough to stop blood circulating past it. This is only applied in the case where bleeding cannot be stopped by any other means and is necessary to prevent the patient from bleeding out.

The base of the skull behind the ears.

**TOURNIQUET**

**Medical Equipment**

# MAXILLA

A device with two rigid poles tied to a fractured leg (or a leg that is suspected to be fractured) with a ratchet at the distal end. A bandage is applied to the ankle and foot and tied to the ratchet. Tension is then applied to realign a broken femur.

The front of the skull.

**TRACTION SPLINT**

Medical Equipment

# ORBITS

A manual or electrically operated pump that creates a suction to withdraw fluids from a patient's trachea and pharynx.

Openings in the anterior skull for the eyeballs.

## SUCTION DEVICE

Medical Equipment

# TEMPORAL

A listening device that allows a provider to hear various sounds within the body for patient assessment, such as the pulse sounds necessary to auscultate blood pressure.

The bones that form the lower sides of the skull.

**STETHOSCOPE**

Medical Equipment

# ZYGOMATIC

Absorbent sterile gauze that is placed directly on open wounds to assist in controled bleeding and in preventing infection.

The cheek bones.

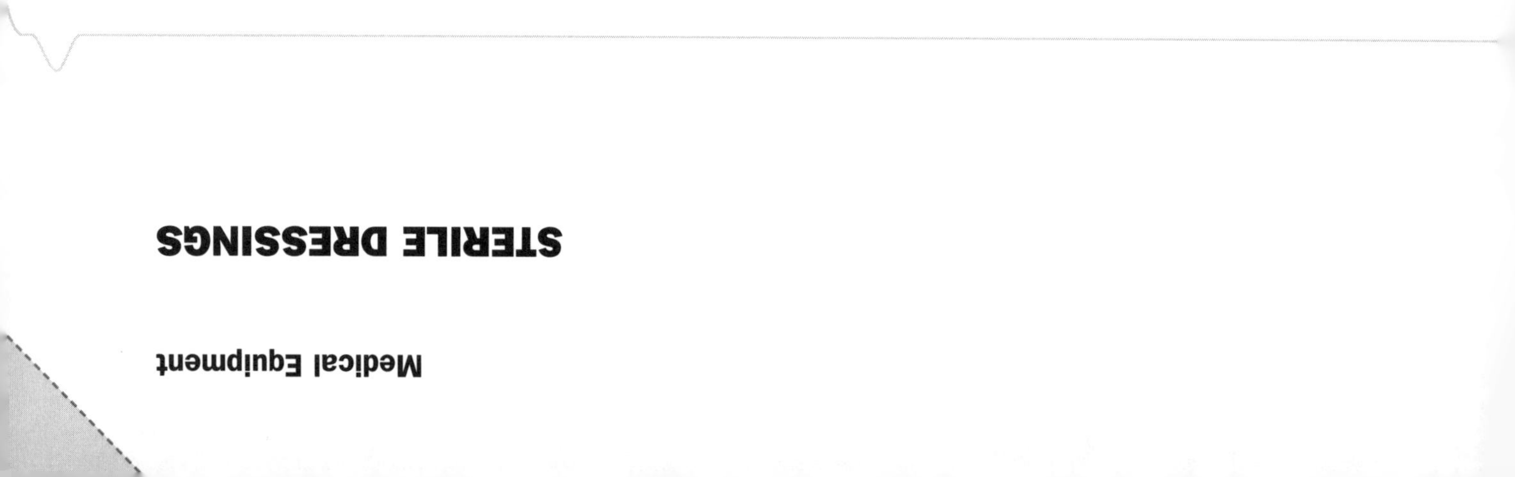

# CERVICAL SPINE

The main stretcher in an ambulance. The stretcher is where the patient sits or lies and is assessed and treated. It accomodates various positions depending on the patient and his or her condition. It is on wheels so that it can be moved easily, especially to relocate a patient.

The top seven vertebrae of the spinal column, which are located in the neck.

**STANDARD STRETCHER**

Medical Equipment

# CLAVICLE

A folding stretcher that allows a patient to be carried in a sitting position up and down stairs. The latest models have tracks on the back that allow a person to be lowered down stair treads without being carried.

Anterior bone connecting the shoulders; the collarbone.

**STAIR CHAIR**

Medical Equipment

# COCCYX

A device that is secured around a patient's upper arm and constricts the brachial artery, stopping blood flow. As it is released, the provider is able to listen for the pulse sound to return, which provides the systolic pressure in millimeters of mercury. Once the pulse sound can no longer be heard, the point on the gauge that corresponds to millimeters of mercury is the diastolic pressure.

The bottom four vertebrae of the spinal column; the tailbone.

**SPHYGMOMANOMETER**

Medical Equipment

# ILIUM

A wood or plastic board designed to be applied just to the torso and head. It can be used to extricate an adult from a vehicle and performs the same function as an extrication vest. It can also be used in the same manner as a long backboard for a child or to provide a firm surface below a patient's torso to perform CPR.

The hip bone.

## SHORT BACKBOARD

Medical Equipment

# LUMBAR SPINE

A cutting tool used to remove clothing from a patient in order to visualize the body for signs and symptoms of illness or injury. Most EMS providers carry heavy duty shears for this with a blunt tip and large plastic handle called "crash scissors."

The five vertebrae between the thoracic and sacral spine; lower back.

**SCISSORS**

Medical Equipment

# PELVIS

A hard plastic tip at the end of the hose leading to the suction unit. Inserted into the pharynx to withdraw fluids. Also known by the brand name "Yankhauer" tip.

The front of the hip bone.

**RIGID SUCTION CATHETER**

Medical Equipment

# RIBS

Padded boards that are tied to a fractured limb (or a limb that is suspected to be fractured) to prevent motion during transport.

A series of bones connected to the sternum and vertebrae that protect the chest and abdominal organs.

**RIGID SPLINTS**

**Medical Equipment**

# SACRAL SPINE (SACRUM)

A two-way communication device carried by an EMS provider to communicate with dispatch and with other members of the crew.

The five vertebrae between the lumbar and coccyx; lower back.

**PORTABLE RADIO**

**Medical Equipment**

# SCAPULA

A simple stretcher made of canvas and two carrying poles. The patient is laid on the canvas and carried to his or her destination.

Flat bones beneath the shoulders on the posterior torso; the shoulder blades.

**POLE STRETCHER**

**Medical Equipment**

A plastic mask carried by many responders to perform artificial ventilation before the arrival of more sophisticated equipment. The mask is applied over a patient's nose and mouth and air is breathed into the patient by the rescuer through a mouthpiece. It is more effective then mouth to mouth resuscitation and safer to the rescuer because it eliminates direct patient contact.

# STERNUM

Anatomy–Bones of the Torso

The bone in the center of the chest to which ribs are connected; the breast bone.

**POCKET MASK**

Medical Equipment

# THORACIC SPINE

The tying of a pillow to a suspected or fractured limb. The pillow has the advantage of being able to be molded into any shape to accommodate the position of the limb.

The seven vertebrae between the cervical and lumbar spine.

**PILLOW SPLINT**

Medical Equipment

# VERTEBRAE

A device that is connected to the oxygen cylinder and releases oxygen at a usable pressure and flow rate.

A series of bones forming the spinal column that allow a person to be upright and that protect the spinal cord.

# OXYGEN REGULATOR

Medical Equipment

# CARPALS

An aluminum, steel, or composite cylinder which stores pure, pressurized oxygen.

The bones of the wrists.

**OXYGEN CYLINDER**

Medical Equipment

# HUMERUS

A rigid, J-shaped tube inserted into the mouth to hold the tongue away from the back of the throat in a deeply unconscious patient. The OPA can only be used if there is no gag reflex in the patient.

The long bone of the upper arm.

**OROPHARYNGEAL AIRWAY (OPA)**

Medical Equipment

# METACARPALS

A type of dressing, usually plastic or vaseline impregnated gauze, that prevents air from entering a wound. This type of dressing is indicated for chest wounds where the lung as been punctured and for neck wounds where air is leaking.

The bones of the hands.

## OCCLUSIVE DRESSINGS

Medical Equipment

# PHALANGES

A prepackaged, sterilized kit of supplies necessary for emergency childbirth delivery. An OB kit will contain sterile gloves, a sterile disposable pad to place beneath the mother's hips, a sterile blanket to place the neonate in to keep it warm, a bulb suction to suction the baby's mouth and nose, sterile sanitary napkins to place over the mother's vagina to control post deliver bleeding, clamps to clamp the umbilical cord, and a sterile scapel or scissors to cut the cord between the clamps.

The bones of the fingers.

**OB KIT**

**Medical Equipment**

# RADIUS

A soft mask and tube with an oxygen reservoir connected to an oxygen regulator and placed over a patient's nose and mouth. It delivers a high concentration of oxygen, typically 80 to 100% of room air.

The medial long bone of the lower arm.

**NON-REBREATHER MASK**

**Medical Equipment**

# ULNA

A flexible tube inserted into the nose to provide a passage for air in a deeply unconscious patient. This device is often used in patients who are having a seizure and have clamped their teeth together.

The lateral long bone of the lower arm.

**NASOPHARYNGEAL AIRWAY**

**Medical Equipment**

# FEMUR

Soft tubing with probes connected to an oxygen regulator that is inserted into a patient's nose and that delivers a low concentration of oxygen, typically 20 to 40% of room air.

The long bone in the upper leg.

## NASAL CANNULA

Medical Equipment

# FIBULA

Disposable coverings for the nose and mouth of the provider to minimize the danger of inhalation of airborne pathogens.

The lateral long bone of the lower leg.

**MASKS**

**Medical Equipment**

# METATARSALS

Plastic devices that are placed over suspected or fractured limbs and then inflated with air to become rigid and prevent motion during transport.

The bones of the feet.

Medical Equipment

## INFLATABLE SPLINTS

Anatomy–Bones of the Legs

# PATELLA

Packages of chemicals that produce warmth when mixed by rupturing the activator inside the primary packaging. These are then placed in the armpits and groin of hypothermic patients to gradually warm them.

The kneecap.

**HEAT PACKS**

**Medical Equipment**

# PHALANGES

A disposable overgarment which protects a provider's clothing from contaminants, primarily blood and bodily fluids.

The bones of the toes.

**GOWNS**

**Medical Equipment**

# TARSALS

Disposable hand coverings which help prevent the spread of infection from patient to provider and vice versa. They were commonly made of latex, but with the increased susceptibility of latex allergies, many services now use non-latex gloves.

The bones of the ankles.

**GLOVES**

Medical Equipment

# TIBIA

Soft plastic tubing at the end of the hose leading to the suction unit. Inserted into the pharynx to withdraw fluids. Also known as a "French" catheter. Used instead of a rigid suction catheter for more gentle suction in less viscous fluid and in pediatric patients.

The meidal long bone of the lower leg.

Medical Equipment

**FLEXIBLE SUCTION CATHETER**

# BRAIN

In addition to its obvious use to illuminate dark areas, a diagnostic flashlight is used to look into the eyes for signs of illness or injury, and to determine the reactivity of the pupils to light, which is an important sign of brain function.

The control center of the certral nervous system. It is responsible for control of all bodily systems.

**FLASHLIGHT**

Medical Equipment

**Anatomy–Organs (Respiratory System)**

# ALVEOLI

Goggles or other devices used to protect the eyes from bodily fluids to minimize the danger of infection from bloodborne or airbone particles.

Sacs at the ends of the bronchioles where oxygen passes into the circulatory system and carbon dioxide is picked up from the circulatory system.

**EYE PROTECTION**

Medical Equipment

# BRONCHUS (PLURAL: BRONCHI)

A rigid device that is strapped on a patient who is entrapped, usually in a wrecked automobile, which allows them to be removed to a standard stretcher while the device minimizes movement of the spinal column to prevent injury to the spinal cord. Also known as a KED (Kendrick Extrication Device).

The tubes leading from the trachea into the bronchioles inside the lungs.

**EXTRICATION VEST**

Medical Equipment

Anatomy–Organs (Respiratory System)

# BRONCHIOLES

A booklet provided by the Department of Transportation that provides listing of all hazardous chemicals transported on the highways with necessary information for EMS providers and firefighters.

The smaller tubes leading from the bronchi to the alveoli.

EMERGENCY RESPONSE GUIDEBOOK

Medical Equipment

Anatomy–Organs (Respiratory System)

# LARYNX

Adhesive pads with conducting gel that are placed on a patient and through which an electrical countershock is applied by an AED (Automated External Defibrillator) or by a manual defibrillator.

The opening in the mouth leading to the throat.

**DEFIBRILLATOR PADS**

Medical Equipment

# LUNGS

Packages of chemicals that produce cold when mixed by rupturing the activator inside the primary packaging. These are then placed in the armpits and groin of hyperthermic patients to gradually coo them. They are also used on injured joints to provide some pain relief and to minimize swelling.

The organs which create negative pressure to bring oxygen into the body and then cycle to positive pressure to expel carbon dioxide from the cellular metabolic process.

**COLD PACKS**

Medical Equipment

**Anatomy–Organs (Respiratory System)**

# TRACHEA

A rigid plastic device that is used to hold the head and neck rigid to minimize the chances of spinal cord damage in a patient with suspected head and neck trauma.

The tube leading from the larynx to the bronchus.

# CERVICAL COLLARS

Medical Equipment

# AORTA

A portable telephone that enables an EMS provider to consult with his or her medical control as well to as notify the receiving facility of their patient's status and condition.

The main artery leading from the heart that carries blood to all other arteries except the pulmonary arteries.

**CELLULAR PHONE**

**Medical Equipment**

# ARTERIOLES

Layers of Kevlar or other material that will prevent the penetration of a projectile or sharp object into the body of a provider. Also known as a bulletproof vest.

The smallest arteries, which link larger arteries to the capillaries.

**BODY ARMOR**

**Medical Equipment**

# AXILLARY ARTERIES

Coverings used to keep patients warm and protect their modesty.

The arteries which carry blood into the arms.

**BLANKETS**

Medical Equipment

# AXILLARY VEINS

Strips of cloth or gauze which are used to secure dressings to wounds.

The veins of the upper arms.

**BANDAGES**

Medical Equipment

Anatomy–Organs (Circulatory System)

# BRACHIAL ARTERIES

A device used to artificially ventilate a patient. The flexible bag is squeezed, forcing air into the mask which is held over the patient's nose and mouth.

The arteries of the upper arm.

**BAG VALVE MASK**

**Medical Equipment**

# CAPILLARIES

A rigid board, usually wood or plastic, upon which a patient can be secured to minimize the danger of unnecessary motion of the spinal column.

The small blood vessels that connect arterioles to the venules and where oxygen passes from the blood to the cells for metabolism.

## BACKBOARD (SPINEBOARD)

Medical Equipment

Anatomy–Organs (Circulatory System)

# CAROTID ARTERIES

A computerized electronic device that analyzes a patient's heart rhythm and delivers a countershock if it detects a correctable dysrhythmia.

The arteries carrying blood from the aorta through the neck to the brain.

## AUTOMATIC EXTERNAL DEFIBRILLATOR (AED)

Medical Equipment

A device with a pre-filled amount of a drug, where the drug can be delivered simply by removing the cap and pushing the injector against a patient. The most common auto injector is the "Epi Pen," which delivers .3 mg of 1:1000 epinephrine in the case of anaphylactic shock.

---

# FEMORAL ARTERIES

**Anatomy–Organs (Circulatory System)**

The arteries of the upper legs.

**AUTO INJECTOR**

**Medical Equipment**

Anatomy–Organs (Circulatory System)

# FEMORAL VEINS

A pediatric patient aged 1 to 3 years of age.

The veins of the mid-leg connecting the tibial veins to the saphenous veins.

**TODDLER**

**Pediatric Terms**

# HEART

A disease which causes apnea and death in infants and toddlers. It is often diagnosed where there is no other explanation for the sudden death of a child.

Two stage, four chambered pump which cirulates blood throughout the body. The four chambers are the right and left atria and the right and left ventricles.

## SUDDEN INFANT DEATH SYNDROME

**Pediatric Terms**

# ILIAC VEINS

A pediatric patient aged 6 to 12 years.

Veins in the pelvic area leading from the legs to the inferior vena cava.

## SCHOOL-AGE CHILD

# INFERIOR VENA CAVA

A pediatric patient aged 3 to 5 years of age.

The inferior vein that carries deoxygenated blood from the lower parts of the body to the heart.

PRE-SCHOOLER

Pediatric Terms

# JUGULAR VEINS

A newborn aged 0 to 30 days.

The veins that carry blood from the brain through the neck back to the superior vena cava.

**NEONATE**

**Pediatric Terms**

# PULMONARY ARTERIES

A pediatric patient aged 1 to 12 months.

The arteries that carry deoxygenated blood from the heart to the lungs.

**INFANT**

**Pediatric Terms**

# PULMONARY VEINS

An unborn child still in his or her mother's uterus. As soon as the fetus is delivered through the vagina he or she becomes a neonate.

The veins carrying oxygenated blood from the lungs to the heart.

**FETUS**

**Pediatric Terms**

Anatomy–Organs (Circulatory System)

# RADIAL ARTERIES

An infection of the epiglottis that mimics the signs and symptoms of croup, but is much more serious and is usually fatal if untreated. Epiglottitis is a true medical emergency and requires the patient to be transported priority to a proper medical facility for treatment.

The arteries of the lower arm.

**EPIGLOTTIS**

**Pediatric Terms**

**Anatomy–Organs (Circulatory System)**

# SAPHENOUS VEINS

A common infection of the upper airway. Croup is characterized by a high pitched barking sound as the patient inhales.

The veins of the upper leg connecting the femoral veins to the iliac veins.

**CROUP**

**Pediatric Terms**

# SUPERIOR VENA CAVA

Situations where a child is not given the normal standards of care in a community. Suspicions of child neglect must be reported to the proper agency by first responders.

The superior vein that leads from the jugular veins into the heart.

**CHILD NEGLECT**

**Pediatric Terms**

# TIBIAL ARTERIES

Situations where a child suffers physical injury by the deliberate act of another. First responders must report any suspicions of child abuse to the proper agency in their jurisdiction.

The arteries of the lower leg.

**CHILD ABUSE**

Pediatric Terms

**Anatomy–Organs (Circulatory System)**

# TIBIAL VEINS

A disease which causes a spasm of the bronchioles and is characterized by a wheezing sound during respirations.

The veins of the lower leg.

**ASTHMA**

**Pediatric Terms**

# VENULES

A pediatric patient between the ages of 12 to 18 years.

The smallest veins, which connect capillaries to larger veins.

**ADOLESCENT**

Pediatric Terms

Anatomy–Organs (Digestive System)

# GALL BLADDER

The level of care that is usual and normal. Deviations from the standard of care may constitute negligence.

The organ where bile, which is produced by the liver, is concentrated and stored. The gall bladder is located in the right upper abdominal quadrant.

**STANDARD OF CARE**

Medical Legal Terminology

# KIDNEYS

A person who experienced a traumatic event such as a sudden death moves back and forth through five different emotional stages; anger, denial, bargaining, depression, and finally acceptance.

The two C shaped organs located in the lower back on either side of the vertebral column. The kidneys filter waste products from the blood in the circulatory system and pass them in the form of urine. The urine passes through the urethras into the urinary bladder, from which it is then voided through the ureter and out through an opening in the genitalia.

**STAGES OF GRIEF**

**Medical Legal Terminology**

Any or a combination of the following may be indicators of severe post-traumatic stress and should be discussed and treated by a mental health professional: sudden irritability, difficulty sleeping, nightmares that awaken, loss of appetite, loss of sexual desire, anxiety, inability to make decisions, spending too much time alone, failure to respond to work when scheduled, and overwheming feelings of guilt.

# LARGE INTESTINE

The part of the intestine from which the products of digestion pass from the small intestine and are further refined into human waste (feces). The large intestine is located in all four abdominal quadrants.

## SIGNS OF POST-TRAUMATIC STRESS

# LIVER

Those specific procedures and protocols permitted to varied levels of licensure. For example an EMT, Basic in most states is permitted to administer epinephrine intramuscular in the event of an allergic reaction, but cannot administer drugs through an intravenous line.

The organ that produces bile (which is used in the digestive process). It is located in the upper right and upper left abdominal quadrants.

**SCOPE OF PRACTICE**

Medical Legal Terminology

# PANCREAS

The first priority of a first responder is to assure his or her own safety and that of the crew with whom he or she is responding. Examples of scenes that are unsafe and must first be made safe include those with violent patients or bystanders, uncontrolled traffic, electrical hazards, and hazardous materials.

An organ that secretes digestive enzymes and hormones, notably insulin used in the breakdown of sugar. The pancreas is located in the lower right and lower left abdominal quadrants.

**SCENE SAFETY**

Medical Legal Terminology

# SMALL INTESTINE

Failure to act as a reasonable and prudent person would under similar circumstances. Negligence is required for a provider to be found liable for injuries.

A long, tubular passage through which disgested food (chyme) is moved, giving off nutrients as it passes along and completing the process of digestion. The small intestine is located in the lower right and lower left abdominal quadrants.

## NEGLIGENCE

**Medical Legal Terminology**

Anatomy–Organs (Digestive System)

# STOMACH

The physician who is the direct overseer of an emergency medical squad and under whose license the squad legally performs medical procedures as allowed by state protocols.

A hollow organ where the main portion of digestion occurs. The stomach is located in the upper left abdominal quadrant.

**MEDICAL DIRECTOR**

Anatomy–Male Reproductive System

# PENIS

---

The physician at a hospital who provides direction and advice to incoming EMS squads. The medical control must also give approval to certain procedures and protocols which can only be performed with the consent of a physician.

The external male sex organ. Semen containing sperm from the testes is ejaculated from its tip into the female vagina to fertilize the female egg, resulting in conception.

**MEDICAL CONTROL**

Medical Legal Terminology

# TESTES

The legal doctrine which presumes that a person unable to give consent would want normal treatment protocols.

Male sex organs that are located in a sac (the scrotum) at the base of the penis in the groin. Sperm manufacturered by the testes are carried by seminal fluid to the tip during sexual arousal.

## IMPLIED CONSENT

Anatomy–Female Reproductive System

# OVARIES

Consent for medical care that is given by a competent patient.

The female sex organs, which are located in the extreme lower abdomen and which carry the eggs. Eggs are released on a monthly cycle through the fallopian tubes. If an egg is fertilized in the tubes, the fertilized egg, now called a zygote, attaches itself to the wall of the uterus and is nourished for the nine month gestation period before delivery.

**EXPRESSED CONSENT**

# UTERUS

The legal doctrine that obliges medical providers to treat and transport patients they encounter.

A hollow organ in the base of the abdomen that receives the zygote and nourishes it for the gestation period. Once the fetus is ready for birth, the uterus begins to contract and pushes the fetus down through the birth canal into the vagina and out.

## DUTY TO ACT

**Medical Legal Terminology**

# VAGINA

A person is competent who is above the age of majority, which is 18 in most states. Competency may also be affected by mental illness or defect and by alcohol or drug intoxication. Only a person who is competent can give assent or refusal of medical treatment.

The opening in the female groin where the male penis is inserted during sexual intercourse. Friction of the penis against the vaginal wall brings about orgasm in the male, with the resultant ejaculation of seminal fluid carrying sperm.

**COMPETENCY**

Anatomy–Skin

# DERMIS

A situation where a medical provider fails in his duty to act and abandons a patient without obtaining proper refusals and releases.

The second layer of skin containing oil and sweat-producing glands.

**ABANDONMENT**

Medical Legal Terminology

**Anatomy–Skin**

# EPIDERMIS

The number of breaths per minute. The normal respiratory rate for infants is 25 to 30 breaths per minute.

The top layer of skin.

**RESPIRATORY RATE**

**Normal Vital Signs–Infant**

# SUBCUTANEOUS TISSUE

The palpable beat resulting from the regular throbbing of blood in the arteries. The normal pulse for an infant is 80 to 140 beats per minute.

The tissue located beneath the two layers of skin.

**PULSE**

**Normal Vital Signs–Infant**

# CARDIAC MUSCLE

Blood pressure is a measure of the force of blood pushing against the walls of the arteries. The normal blood pressure for infants is 70 to 100 mm of mercury (Hg). The first number is the systolic blood pressure, or the pressure when the ventricles are contracting; the second number is the diastolic blood pressure, or the pressure when the ventricles are at rest.

The type of muscle that is responsible solely for the pumping action of the heart.

**BLOOD PRESSURE**

Normal Vital Signs–Infant

# SKELETAL MUSCLE

The number of breaths per minute; the normal respiratory rate for children ranges from 15 to 30 breaths per minute.

The tissues that are responsible for the movement of the body and its parts by expanding and contracting.

**RESPIRATORY RATE**

**Normal Vital Signs–Pediatric**

Anatomy–Muscle

# SMOOTH

The palpable beat resulting from the regular throbbing of blood in the arteries. The normal pulse for a child is 70 to 110 beats per minute.

Tissues that are not connected to the skeleton and that cause motion, such as digestion, reproduction and waste elimination.

**PULSE**

**Normal Vital Signs–Pediatric**

Blood pressure is a measure of the force of blood pushing against the walls of the arteries. The normal blood pressure for children is 80 to 120 mm of mercury (Hg). The first number is the systolic blood pressure, or the pressure when the ventricles are contracting; the second number is the diastolic blood pressure, or the pressure when the ventricles are at rest.

# BLOOD PRESSURE

Blood pressure is a measure of the force of blood pushing against the walls of the arteries. The normal blood pressure for adults is 120 to 80 mm of mercury (Hg). The first number is the systolic blood pressure, or the pressure when the ventricles are contracting; the second number is the diastolic blood pressure, or the pressure when the ventricles are at rest.

# BLOOD PRESSURE

Normal Vital Signs–Pediatric

Normal Vital Signs–Adult

# PULSE

The number of breaths per minute; the normal respiratory rate for adults ranges from 12 to 16 respirations per minute.

The palpable beat caused by the regular throbbing in the arteries that is caused by the contractions in the heart. The normal pulse for an adult is 68 to 74 beats per minute.

## RESPIRATORY RATE

Normal Vital Signs–Adult

# ABOUT THE AUTHOR

**Richard J. Lapierre** is the Director of Emergency Medical Services for Brown University, which provides pre-hospital Advanced Life Support service and transport to the campus community, as well as Basic and Advanced EMT courses. He is a licensed Emergency Medical Technician, Cardiac and an EMS Instructor/Coordinator for the state of Rhode Island. He is also a retired Deputy Fire Chief from the Oakland-Mapleville (RI) Fire Department. In addition, he is an emergency telecommunicator for the Burrillville (RI) Police Department, where he also serves as chaplain and one of the SRT Medics. He holds a Bachelor of Science degree from the University of Rhode Island and a Master of Arts degree from Providence College. He is the author of the Kaplan guide fo the EMT-Basic Exam.